# Detox
# LIVER AND GALLBLADDER DETOX
*Natural Body Cleanse*

By Jennifer Atkins

2nd Edition

© Copyright 2014 - All rights reserved.

In no way is it legal to reproduce, duplicate, or transmit any part of this document in either electronic means or in printed format. Recording of this publication is strictly prohibited and any storage of this document is not allowed unless with written permission from the publisher. All rights reserved.

The information provided herein is stated to be truthful and consistent, in that any liability, in terms of inattention or otherwise, by any usage or abuse of any policies, processes, or directions contained within is the solitary and utter responsibility of the recipient reader. Under no circumstances will any legal responsibility or blame be held against the publisher for any reparation, damages, or monetary loss due to the information herein, either directly or indirectly.

Respective authors own all copyrights not held by the publisher.

Legal Notice:

This ebook is copyright protected. This is only for personal use. You cannot amend, distribute, sell, use, quote or paraphrase any part or the content within this ebook without the consent of the author or copyright owner. Legal action will be pursued if this is breached.

Disclaimer Notice:

Please note the information contained within this document is for educational and entertainment purposes only. Every attempt has been made to provide accurate, up to date and reliable complete information. No warranties of any kind are expressed or implied. Readers acknowledge that the author is not engaging in the rendering of legal, financial or professional advice.

By reading this document, the reader agrees that under no circumstances are we responsible for any losses, direct or indirect, which are incurred as a result of the use of information contained within this document, including, but not limited to, —errors, omissions, or inaccuracies

# Table of Contents

Introduction

Chapter 1- The Anatomy Of The Liver

Chapter 2- Functions Of The Liver

Chapter 3- What Is Detoxification?

Chapter 4- The Alarming Symptoms Of Liver Toxicity

Chapter 5- Various Benefits Of Liver Detoxification

Chapter 6: Foods That Enhance Liver Detox

Chapter 7: Design Your Own Diet Plan For Detox

Chapter 8: Refreshing Juice Recipes

Chapter 9: Healthy Salad Recipes

Chapter 10: Soups

Chapter 11: Exercise And Yoga For Liver Cleanse

Chapter 12: Foods To Avoid

Conclusion

# Introduction

Each and every part of the human body serves a specific purpose. The brain serves the purpose of thought generation while the heart serves the purpose of pumping blood. The kidney functions by cleansing the blood and the intestines digest food.

Similarly, the liver works by breaking down the food that we consume, convert it into energy and stores it for later use.

It is therefore one of the most important organ in the body and maintaining a clean liver will help us lead a long healthy life.

But given our hectic lifestyles and excessive dependence on junk food, our liver is most affected. Various factors such as medications, viruses, alcohol consumption etc. cut down on our liver's capacity to function optimally.

It is therefore important to understand the various foods we must consume to strengthen it, the exercises that we must do to promote its good health and also have a look at the various foods and beverages that one must avoid while on the liver cleansing diet.

In this book, we explore all the above mentioned aspects in detail and help guide you towards attaining a clean and healthy liver. I thank you for downloading this eBook and hope for it to act as your one true "Liver Detox" guide.

# Chapter 1- The Anatomy Of The Liver

***What is the liver?***

The liver is the largest gland in the body, contributing to about two percent of the total body weight. In an adult, the average liver weighs about 3 pounds or 1.5 kilograms. After the skin, the liver is the largest organ of the body and is shaped like a wedge.

The liver is soft and pliable and occupies the upper part of the abdominal cavity, just beneath the diaphragm, within the rib cage in the upper right quadrant of the abdomen. The liver is so big that it spans across the right hypochondria region, the epigastria and a part of the left hypochondriac region. The liver is generally reddish brown in color. The red color is due to the excess blood that the liver contains throughout the day, which darkens after the consumption of food.

The liver may be divided into a large right lobe and a small left lobe. The right lobe is further divided into a quadrate lobe and a caudate lobe by the presence of the gallbladder. Anatomically, the quadrate lobe and the caudate lobe are a part of the right lobe of the liver, but physiologically these lobes are a part of the left lobe. The right lobe is at least 6 times larger than the left lobe, which causes the liver to have an asymmetric shape. The liver has a sharp inferior border.

It also contains 3 lobules, with each one serving a different purpose. The first one being the classical lobule whose main purpose is to hold the entire structure of the liver together. The second is the portal lobule whose main activity involves the secretion of the important bile liquid that is used to digest and break down food. The third section is the Acinus that is responsible for the regulation of blood flow and the metabolic activity.

The liver has five surfaces:

1. superior surface
2. anterior surface
3. posterior surface
4. inferior surface
5. right surface

Men on an average have larger livers than women.

The blood vessels conveying blood to the liver are the hepatic artery and the portal vein. The function of the hepatic artery is to bring oxygenated blood to the liver, and the function of the portal vein is to bring in venous blood. Both, the arterial blood and the venous blood are conducted to the central vein.

The liver produces a large amount of lymph, about one third to half of all body lymph. Lymph is said to be the liquid that flows through the lymphatic system, and aids in returning the extra interstitial fluid and the protein back into circulation.

The lymph vessels leave the liver and enter several lymph nodes in the porta hepatitis, which is a short fissure present in the liver.

## *Anatomy of the Gall Bladder*

The gallbladder is a small pear shaped sac, lying on the surface of the liver. It has a capacity to easily contain 30 to 50 ml of liquid, and stores bile, which it concentrates by absorbing water.

The gallbladder is divided into 3 parts: the fundus, the body and the neck.

# Chapter 2- Functions Of The Liver

The liver performs many different functions, and many of its functions interrelate with one another. The liver has several functions that it needs to perform on a daily basis, in order to keep a person fit and healthy.

The functions can be divided as follow:

- Bile production and secretion
- Nutrient absorption
- Storage
- Cleansing
- Balancing chemical levels
- Glucose dissemination

## *Bile Production and Secretion*
One of the main purposes of the liver is the secretion of bile, which is usually between 600 ml to 1000 ml per day. The bile is a liquid that is produced in the bile duct and helps in the breaking down of the fats in the intestines.

The liquid varies in color, depending on the person's health and his or her food habits, and ranges between dark green and yellowish brown.

Although the liver produces the bile, the bile does not stay there and rapidly travels to the gall bladder, which is where the bile is stored. The bladder then releases the bile into the stomach every time you consume food that contains fats. The liquid then immediately gets to work and starts to break down the fat cells.

No other part of the body can produce the bile liquid, apart from the liver.

### *Nutrient Absorption*

The liver acts like a sponge, which absorbs both nutrients and toxins and breaks them down as per their value. That is to say, the liver absorbs the nutrients, breaks them down into molecules that are most beneficial for the body, and helps in transporting these molecules to where they are required the most.

At the same time, they also absorb the toxins and break them down to molecules that pose least risk to the body. This process is known as Detoxification.

The nutrients and toxins undergo a dual screening, where they first get broken down in the intestines, and then travel to the liver for further breakdown.

All types of food nutrients and toxins pass through the liver, including solid food, liquids, and medicines.

### *Storage*

The liver acts like a storage unit for several nutrients. Some of these nutrients are good for the whole body, while some are vital for the smooth functioning of the liver.

The various nutrients stored in the liver include iron, copper, and vitamins - A, D, E, K, and B12.

At any given time, the liver has a reserve of the aforementioned nutrients that it keeps ready to be transported to the various organs of the body, if the need may be.

## *Cleansing*

The liver purifies the blood that passes through it. It acts like a sponge that absorbs all the toxins and the blood that leaves the liver is extremely clean and pure. It also helps in the process of blood clots and keeps a reserve of blood that it secretes when the body needs it.

## *Balancing Chemical Levels*

The liver helps in balancing the chemical levels in the blood by trying to break down the harmful toxins as much as possible.

It also helps balance the hormones in the body and is especially important for women. The liver helps produce serum proteins, which act as hormone carriers. It also helps produce the testosterone in men and estrogen in women and also helps in balancing out the sex hormones in the body.

## *Glucose Dissemination*

The liver absorbs all the blood that passes through the walls of the intestines and contains quite a bit of carbohydrates. The liver absorbs the carbohydrates and converts them to glycogen. Glycogen is a simplified form of glucose, which the liver then converts to glucose and transports into the blood stream whenever you require some energy to do any task.

## *Immunity*

Immunity and the liver go hand in hand. Gamma globulin is a substance that is essential in building immunity and is produced and secreted by the liver.

The liver contains cells called the Kupffer cells, whose main function is to absorb various bacteria, viruses, fungi, and other parasites that can cause diseases in the body.

The liver works at a very fast pace to quickly absorb the blood and allow the Kupffer cells to go through every ounce of blood and get rid of all the parasites and other substances, such as defunct blood cells and cell debris.

It is, therefore, extremely crucial to help keep the liver functioning to its full capacity, in order to keep the body fit and healthy.

# Chapter 3- What Is Detoxification?

Detoxification is the process of removing toxins or unwanted material from the organs of a living organism. By detoxification the body reaches a state of neutralization. The process can be self-induced and is meant to help the body clean itself internally. It is truly said, *"You are what you eat"*. Out of all the organs of the body, the liver is the most stressed organ because it is responsible for performing various functions, all alone, to keep the body fit and healthy. Liver is the whole and sole filtering machine of your body and without it the body wouldn't be able to repel and filter the toxins from the body.

We are all aware of the importance external cleanliness that has been taught to us in school. We bathe every day, wash our hair every day and brush our teeth twice a day; in short, we all like to look good and smell good. But, detoxification is the inner cleanliness of the body, which helps us to eliminate all the dangerous toxins and sadly, not a lot of us do enough for our internal cleanliness, as we do for out external cleanliness.

Almost all organs in the body can and should be detoxed on a regular basis, but the most important organ that requires regular detoxification is the liver.

The liver is responsible for several functions in the body. As was seen in chapter 3, the liver performs numerous activities that help keep the body healthy.

But, the liver can be a little sensitive and over the years, by doing such important services to keep the human body healthy, it starts to deteriorate and slowdown in its functioning, owing to several factors.

These factors are introduced into the body mostly through the consumption of harmful food and exposure to parasites. The liver might also absorb impurities from the air and the various harmful chemicals that are employed on a daily basis.

Once the liver starts to deteriorate, it becomes quite difficult to put it back on the right track. However, it is possible for the liver to regenerate itself, and it also has the capacity to adjust its size as per the person's body requirements. The liver is known for it to be medically possible for a healthy liver to lose up to 55% of its volume, and yet regenerate to 100% within one to one and a half months' time.

Detoxification should be done at two levels, dietary changes as well as lifestyle changes. Both these changes go hand in hand, and it helps us decrease the intake of toxins, and helps in rapid elimination of the toxins, if any.

It is, however, extremely important to keep the liver clean and undergo a cleansing routine from time to time. Because when cleansing of the liver is delayed by even a few days or months, it can be extremely harmful to the body. It also makes it difficult to maintain a proper balance between all the organs, thus destroying the harmony. If the toxin stays in your body for a long period of time, it can putrefy and even be reabsorbed by the body, thus becoming a major breeding ground for serious diseases.

It is a good idea to cleanse your body once or twice a year. Detoxification is like resetting your body all over again. Detoxification not only improves your physical health, but it also improves your state of mind. Detoxifying your body boosts you up with extra energy, helps you in balancing and regulating the important hormones, improves digestion and assimilation, beautifies your skin and also makes you feel happy.

Many of these toxins come from the food we consume or the diet that we follow on regular basis, the unnecessary drugs that we swallow, and also the environment. The toxins need to be flushed out and this can be done through the consumption of the right types of foods and liquids.

It can also be done by employing an effective exercise regimen and the use of alternate therapy like yoga.

Another method is to undergo cleansing surgeries and processes such as liver and colon cleanses.

# Chapter 4- The Alarming Symptoms Of Liver Toxicity

Liver toxicity is the internal derangement of the body. But yes, it does manifest its symptoms on the physical level as well as the mental level. So it is very necessary to know the alarming symptoms.

## *Lack of Concentration*

Due to the excessive amount of toxins that are being circulated in the blood, there is a noticeable decrease in concentration levels. The individual is not capable of focusing on a particular thing and may find themselves zoning out quite frequently. You may notice this symptom quite late, because we all feel that it is may be due to stress or something else, but most of the times you never guess that it can be due to the excessive amounts of toxins in your blood.

## *Easily Fatigued*

These days many individuals complaint of getting fatigued quite easily, where in they may experience a lack of energy to do tasks or experience a complete loss of energy. After doing little amounts of work, they may experience a decrease in energy levels, and so to meet the energy needs they sip stimulants like caffeine. Stimulants definitely help them compensate that lack of energy, and they are able to work for hours after that. But, what we forget is the toxins that we ingest to fulfill our energy needs. There are people who do not wake up fresh in the morning and feel sluggish all through the day. These are the individuals who need to undergo a detox, in order to dispel the harmful toxins that prevent the liver from producing and storing energy.

## *Struggling With Weight Loss*

Losing weight is a difficult and energy consuming journey, but being healthy is the shining trophy at the end of the road, and the effort and aches you put in are completely worth the end result. Achieving health and fitness is not a destination; it is a way of life in order to achieve a better living. You may come across many hurdles when you are trying hard to lose those extra flabs, and these pent up toxins in your body can be the main cause for the difficulty to lose weight. Detox helps you in removing those extra toxins from your body and further helps you to shed weight.

## *Skin Problems*

There may have been times when you may have faced skin problems, and you had visited the best doctor in town, tried and experimented with the most expensive lotions and therapies, but nothing worked in clearing your sin up. Skin problems also arise due to excess of toxicity in the body, which manifests itself on the surface of the skin as a rash or a pimple. When you know the basic cause of a problem, it makes it easier to treat and heal it. Detox helps in treating this root cause and results in a glowing and smooth skin in no time at all.

## *Sleep Disorders*

Excessive toxins in your body can disturb and change your sleeping patterns. You may be awake all night, turning and tossing in your bed. Due to lack of appropriate night sleep, your natural cycle is hampered, which further destroys your everyday routine cycle. Since you do not get sound sleep in the night, you tend to get up late in the mornings, resulting in a vicious cycle of late mornings and even later nights. Detoxifying the body provides you with a natural, restful and sound sleep, and ensures that you wake up fresh in the morning.

## *Digestion Problems*

Constipation is a very common problem in this decade. There are many people who suffer from chronic constipation. If you have tried things like increasing your water intake, increasing your intake of fibrous food and also changing your eating habits, but still you are struggling with hard stools and incomplete evacuation, you need to realize that your body is screaming for a detox. The detox will help you clean and free your body from stored up fecal matter and toxins, and the detox also promotes proper digestion, absorption and assimilation.

## *Feeling Depressed*

Have you ever heard that an individual's mood is influenced a lot by what he or she eats? It is largely believed that what you feel and the mood that you are in depends on what type of food you consume on an everyday basis. It is very important to eat the right food, essential for proper growth and good health. Unhealthy food provides you with only empty calories and is full of toxins. Eating healthy and right boosts your energy and makes you feel joyous and happy.

## *Negativity*

Healthy eating is also the key to proper and clear thinking and brings positivity in life. There are times when your mind has no capacity left to think. The toxins in your body block your capacity to think, which is required for correct and reasonable thinking. What you think of is all the negative aspects of life and the positivity is lost. A negative mind is the worst thing to have, because it will only put you in to depression and nothing else. Detox your body, it will not only clear up the toxins, but also give you a chance to look at life in a different and more positive way.

## *Sexual Dysfunction*

A lot of individuals complain of decreased or loss of sexual drive and sexual power or even complaint of insufficient performance. Excessive toxins in the system could be the major cause behind this. Your body needs to balance the hormonal levels in correct proportions in order for the arousal of the sexual desire in you, and the toxins can act as a hurdle in regulating hormonal levels in the body. Research has shown that people who have under gone a detox session have a stronger sexual drive and a better performance in the sack. Sometimes, people think that decreased sexual desire could be a sign of ageing, but all you need is to detox yourself and see the difference.

# Chapter 5- Various Benefits Of Liver Detoxification

The benefits of liver detox are very many. They are categorized as follows:

- Eliminating Gallstones
- Improving digestion
- Helping with weight loss
- Clearing up the skin
- Regulating hormonal balance
- Bettering immunity
- Controlling sugar levels
- Improving mental ability

### *Eliminating Gallstones*
When the liver produces bile, it is transported and stored in the gall bladder. Sometimes, the liver starts to develop stones that

either stay behind and block the bile ducts or move to the bladder and interrupt its smooth functioning.

When these stones block the bile duct, adequate bile does not get secreted and the liver is forced into overdrive. When it works too hard, it starts to lose some vigor and the body starts to develop various illnesses. Also, when these stones are stuck in the bladder, they make it painful to pass urine and cause immense amounts of pain. It is, therefore, important to flush out gallstones.

### *Improving Digestion*

The liver filters and digests several fats and other substances that are not broken down by the kidneys. The bile that is secreted by the liver helps in breaking down all types of substances, including nutrients and toxins and other complex substances.

When fats are broken down, the body easily absorbs them. The liver also helps in easing bowel movement and aids in maintaining a healthy metabolism level.

### *Helping With Weight Loss*

According to several researchers and medical practitioners, obese people generally have a malfunctioning liver, which causes their bodies to store irregular amounts of fat. The liver is responsible for metabolizing and digesting fats. The liver produces and stores bile and this bile helps in the breakdown of fat. There are people who struggle with unhealthy diets and unhealthy lifestyles that result in fullness, heaviness, gastric problems and weight gain. It is, therefore, extremely crucial to cleanse the liver from time to time to ensure that the storage of fat in the body as per the requirement of the body and not extra.

The cleansing routine will help eradicate the root cause of weight gain, especially in the stomach region, and not allow the body to gain back the weight that it loses.

### *Clearing Up The Skin*

The skin is a true indicator of the internal state of affairs of a person and any problem inside will almost always have a bearing on the outside.

When the liver contains a backlog of excessive waste, such as toxins and other bodily wastes, the skin starts to erupt with zits and acne, and also starts to lose elasticity due to the breaking down of the collagen. This is why it is important to maintain a clean liver that is free from toxins and free radicals in order to have a flawless and clean skin.

### *Regulating Hormonal Balance*

Several hormone related diseases, such as PCOD (polycystic ovarian disease), and other common illnesses can be regulated by the cleansing of the liver.

The liver produces and helps balance the various hormones required to keep the endocrine system functioning smoothly.

If the liver is overloaded with toxins, it loses its capacity to produce the right amount of hormones and also fails to produce the carriers that carry these hormones to the right parts of the body.

### *Better Immunity*

The liver contains Kupffer cells, which form the first line of defense against disease causing pathogens. These cells absorb the various parasites that enter the body's blood stream and cause it to develop various diseases.

It also absorbs the various chemicals and toxins that enter the body through various orifices, such as the nostrils and the mouth, and does not allow them to enter the blood stream.

Therefore, by keeping the liver clean, a person can boost their levels of immunity.

### Controlling Sugar Levels

The liver has the capacity of absorbing excessive glucose and converting it into glycogen, which it stores for later use. It more or less prevents insulin malfunction by absorbing excessive sugar and only releases it when the body needs energy.

With the regulated amounts of sugar levels, the body reduces the risk of developing diabetes, and the person experiences regulated levels of energy.

### Improving Mental Ability

One of the main functions of the brain is to convert ammonia into urea. This is because when ammonia reaches the brain, it causes it to slow down. Urea on the other hand does not slow down brain function and it also helps in the reduction of headaches.

## Chapter 6: Foods That Enhance Liver Detox

Is it possible to enjoy a food plan which features liver purifying food products, without starving yourself or transforming your regular scheduled day plan? Research has verified that by incorporating the foods that are going to provide us with detox characteristics, anyone can follow this regimen, and attain the best benefits out of it. When it comes to detox the liver, a person can follow a strict diet regimen, which allows the consumption of only those foods that help in effectively flushing out the various toxins that can build up over a period of time.

So what are these food products, and how hard is it going to be for us to include these foods in our regular weekly eating plan? It is going to be a little difficult initially, but as time passes an individual will be used to it, because the end result is being healthy, which is the major priority for all. You will notice that these food products are abundant with minerals, vitamins, dietary fibers and antioxidants. Additionally, they will be no problem by any means fitting these food products into your every week diet plan.

Here, we highlight the various foods and also explain their contents, which help in the process of detox.

## *Solid foods*

### Beetroots

Loaded with beta-carotene and iron, beetroots are regarded as the number one foods to consume in order to cleanse the liver. Beetroots also contains essential anti oxidants, which slow down the oxidation with other molecular components.

Beetroot when consumed help in production of glutathione in the body. Glutathione is a natural detoxifying agent, which helps in eliminating the stored toxins in the body.

Beetroots are also rich in Betaine. Research has proved that Betaine is a very important compound for the liver to function properly. Betaine promotes in regeneration of the liver cells, and also increases the production of bile, which improves the livers capacity to eliminate toxins faster.

Beetroot is not only a good detoxifier, but it helps in shedding of those extra weigh, prevents aging and improves digestion.

Consuming half a raw beetroot in the form of a salad ingredient or even having one glass of fresh beetroot juice can go a long way in cleaning your liver and keeping it healthy. You can also consume beetroot in juice form or even cooked, but make sure you don't overcook them, because by doing that they lose their healthy properties.

### Eggs

Eggs are rich in quality proteins. They contain all the eight essential amino acids that are necessary for detoxifying the body. Choline is a coenzyme present in the egg yolk, which helps in protecting the liver from further damage. Egg also helps in improving the metabolism of the body.

## Berries

Strawberries, blueberries, raspberries and cranberries they are all super foods. These berries contain polyphenols and anthocyanins, which protects the liver from cancer.

## Onions

Onions are found in most kitchens. They are rich in sulfur rich amino acids, which are essential for liver detox. It also contains quercetin and anthocyanins, which absorbs all the unwanted toxins from the body. Onions contain potassium, phytonutrients and flavanoids, which help the body to fight various disease conditions, thus improving the immune system. Onions are best consumed raw, or they can also be added in curries and stews by making their paste.

## Garlic

Garlic is a super food and is not needed in a large amount to activate the liver enzymes, it not just helps in cleaning your liver but also aids in its optimal functioning. Just by placing a pod of garlic under your tongue that's sliced in half will help draw out all the toxins from the liver and also activate its various enzymes. It also contains allicin and selenium, which help in cleaning the liver naturally.

## Artichokes

Artichokes contain a substance called cynarin and silymarin, which helps in stimulating the functions of the liver and the gallbladder. They also help in cleansing the kidneys. Artichokes also help in preventing gallstones.

Steamed and roasting artichokes are the best way to consume them. Artichokes can also be eaten raw by adding them in salad along with your favorite dressing.

## Ginger

Ginger comes from the roots. It is that food product which our ancient civilization has used profusely, as it is believed to have many medicinal properties. Ginger also has some astringent properties that help the liver function properly. It is very useful for people who are diagnosed with fatty liver, due to excess of alcohol intake.

You can add ginger in your daily refreshing drinks or even in your tea. Ginger can also be consumed in hot water. You can also cook it, by adding it into your meals, and giving your palate a different taste.

**Green leafy vegetables**
The functioning of green leafy vegetables inside the body can be compared with their functioning in their natural habitat. Just like green leaves help absorb the toxins in the environment, they help in absorbing the toxins from the liver. They have the capacity to neutralize the harmful chemicals, thus working hard as the best filtering machine for flushing out toxins from the body.

The leaves are full of plant chlorophyll, which helps in the process of absorption of toxins and the leaves can be consumed in any form including cooked, raw and juiced.

**Cabbage and lettuce**
Cabbage and lettuce both help the liver activate two main enzymes that are needed by the liver to function optimally. Cabbage also helps the liver to lower your cholesterol and so this cruciferous vegetable is very important for you to include in your diet. Also cabbage increases our urine output, thus helping to eliminate all the extra toxins out of the body.

It is therefore important to snack on cabbage and lettuce as much as possible and they are best eaten raw in the form of salad ingredients after being thoroughly cleansed under running water.

**Bitter gourd**
The bitter gourd is horrible to taste but is loaded with nutrients that aid in the cleansing of the liver. It is full of vitamin C, which

helps in flushing out the toxins in the blood even before it reaches the kidney. It thereby cuts down on the workload of the kidneys.

## Tomatoes

Tomatoes contain the chemical glutathione, which help in detoxifying liver. They also contain the flavanoids called lycopene, which help combat the free radicals and help prevent liver cancer. They are best eaten raw with a little serving of sea salt sprinkled on top.

## Broccoli

Broccoli is a superfood that helps the body in many ways. One of its main uses is in the treating of livers that are flooded with toxins. Rich in sulfurophane, broccoli helps in flushing out the toxins from the liver. Broccoli can be eaten raw or juiced or made into a soup. It is better absorbed in the liquid form.

## Asparagus

A natural diuretic, the asparagus helps the liver in converting ammonia into urea. It also helps clean the liver and eliminate toxins. Asparagus also helps the liver in drainage, since the liver is responsible to filter out the food we consume, it helps to pick up those toxic material, and helps elimination. Asparagus also has anti-aging and anti-inflammatory properties, and protects you from cancer.

Asparagus can be eaten raw or cooked. It is best eaten par boiled and eaten as an evening snack. It also helps clean the stomach clean and does not allow toxins to pass through to the liver.

## Lemons and limes

Lemon ranks first in detoxifying the body. Lemons and limes contain extremely high levels of vitamin c, which is crucial in breaking down toxins, which can be harmful for the body. Lemons also have high level of citric acid that helps in improving digestion. Lemon also helps in cleansing the bowels, by eliminating the waste from our body. Lemon also helps in excess secretion of bile, which in turn helps in detoxification.

The vitamin c helps in breaking down the toxins, which is easily absorbed by water. Few drops of lemon in lukewarm water in the morning, is highly recommended for detox plan. You can also include lemons in your salad dressing, giving it an extra punch and tanginess.

## Peppermint

This mint is very famous for refreshing the oral cavity, which results in fresh breath. Peppermint helps to detoxify the liver by relaxing the bile ducts and stimulating the flow of bile. Mint helps in reducing the bad cholesterol from the body, thus making it faster and easier for the liver to filter and eliminate all the toxins from the body. Peppermint also helps in improving digestion by removing any blockages from the gall bladder and the kidney, if any.

## Whole grains

Whole grains contain B-complex vitamins that help in the breaking down of fats. Therefore, whole grains, such as brown rice and whole wheat flour, help the liver function better. They make for great substitutes for white flour and other grains that contain gluten.

## Avocados

Avocados are the best fruits to consume in order to cleanse the liver. They are full of glutathione, which help flush out the toxins from the liver. They also aid the liver in flushing out the toxins from the blood.

Avocados can be eaten alone without any other ingredient for getting their full benefit, or you can even enjoy it by adding it to your smoothie along with papaya and strawberries.

## Grape fruit

Grape fruits are loaded with vitamin c, which helps flush out toxins. They can be eaten or juiced and help in fighting away carcinogens and help boost the immune system. Grape fruit helps in burning up the fats and so it is a well proven fruit for weight loss. Grape fruit prepares your liver to be active and take proper action, against the toxins.

## Apples

Apples contain pectin, which helps in eliminating the toxins from the digestive tract. By doing so, apples help in cutting down on the load that is taken on by the liver. Apples also contain malic acid, which helps in eliminating the carcinogens from the body. They are also a great source of anti-oxidants. Apples also help the liver flush out their toxins and an apple every morning will help in easing bowel movement. Try to consume apples that are organic, do not opt for apples which are sprayed with pesticides, they are a burden to your liver.

## Walnuts

Walnuts contain an amino acid called arginine, which helps in the breaking down and elimination of ammonia. Since the liver helps break down ammonia and convert them to urea, walnuts aid livers in the very process. They also contain omega 3 fatty acids, which help in the cleansing of the liver. A handful of walnuts make a good snack.

## Carrots

Carrots are rich in beta-carotene, which help in the cleansing of the liver. They help cleaning out the toxins, which might cause a person to develop skin problems such as zits and pimples. Carrots also help improve the eyesight, by providing sufficient vitamin A, to the body thus curing various eye related problems. They are best eaten raw and sliced into juliennes so that they are easily broken down.

## Turmeric

Turmeric is extensively used in Indian and other Asian cuisines as a spice, for their anti-carcinogenic properties. It is especially used in the cleansing of the liver as it activates the enzymes that are important in helping the liver function optimally. Turmeric is also a great anti septic. You can include turmeric in your detox diet by adding it into your tea. They almost immediately help in flushing out the toxins and parasites from the liver.

## Yogurt

Yogurt is on the top list, if you wish to have effective and smooth digestion. The good bacteria that is essential for our body's, which helps in breakdown of food, helps in digestion and immune system, and is provided by yogurt. Yogurt also fills up your stomach fast, avoiding excess unwanted eating, and thus aids in weight loss. Snack on yogurt with some chopped fresh fruits, whenever you are hungry. It is also a great source of protein. Yogurt also contains enough calcium, preventing bone related diseases.

## Cauliflower

Cauliflower also belongs to the cruciferous group. Cauliflowers are a good source of vitamin C and vitamin K. Vitamin K protects the liver from getting damaged, and also if the damage to the liver has happened it helps to restore and regenerate the liver quickly. Cauliflower can be eaten raw as a salad with dressing, or one can even boil, sauté and puree this nutritious vegetable.

## Milk thistle

Milk thistle contains a component silymarin, which acts as a natural liver protector. It is also used for treating diseases that occur due to excess drinking of alcohol like acute and chronic hepatitis. It has been discovered that the major health benefit is obtained by using highly concentrated thistle extract, which contains 80% of standardized silymarin in it. Silymarin is also a very essential compound for promoting liver cell regeneration, preventing further damage. It helps in slowing down the process of irreversible liver damage in patients who are diseased due to alcohol abuse. It is also a good source of antioxidants.

## Hemp seeds

Hemp seeds have gained a lot of attention recently due to their immense positive effects on the body. Hemp seeds contain all the essential amino acids, which are required for the body to function properly. It contains a balanced amount of omega 6 and omega 3 fatty acids, which are the good type of fats that helps in metabolizing the fats in the liver and reduces the risk of cholesterol. Intake of hemp seeds on regular basis helps in improving the defense mechanism of the body.

## Chia seeds

These seeds come under the category of super food. It is a member of the mint family, but tastes completely different from the mint; its taste is neutral on the palate. Chia seeds are high in fiber, which helps in improving digestion and bowel movements. It contains certain essential amino acids, which the body is unable to produce on its own, and needs to get from the food that we eat. Chia seeds are also high in anti-oxidants, potassium, iron and calcium and helps in fulfilling the everyday need of the body.

Chia seeds can be consumed in the morning, after soaking them in water for 30 minutes. You can even sprinkle these small seeds full of proteins in your smoothies and other preparations.

## Flax seeds

Flax seeds are a healthy food for the liver. They contain alpha linolenic acid or ALA, known precursor of omega 3 fatty acids, which helps in balancing the cholesterol levels in the body. This ALA also helps in reducing the inflammation in the liver caused by the toxins, and inhibits cellular damage. Flax seeds are also high in soluble and insoluble type of fiber that can help in easy digestion and can boost the metabolic activity of the body. It is also a leading therapy to cure fatty liver disease. Flax seeds can be used in various juices and smoothies as a topping; it enhances the flavor of the drink by giving it a nutty texture.

## *Liquid foods*

### Water

Water is one of the most important of liquids that is used in the process of detoxification, either of the liver or any organ of the body. Hydrating yourself is very important, especially if you are working out daily, since you lose a lot of water in the form of sweat. Water helps collect all the toxins that are water-soluble and gets rid of it in the form of sweat and urine.

If you cannot drink large quantity of water at a time, make sure you have at least 1 glass, every hour. It is therefore mandatory to drink at least 10-12 glasses of water a day and a popular diet known as the water diet is used to help clean the liver naturally. Increased water intake is the best way one can get rid of toxins.

### Green tea

Green tea has gained a lot of popularity in this decade, because of its benefits on the health. Green tea contains a type of anti-oxidant, called polyphenol, which helps in flushing out toxins from the body. Research has been made that it also contains a substance called catechins, which protect the liver from getting damaged and also improves the liver functions. It also helps in losing weight, by boosting up the metabolic activity. Full of anti-oxidants, green tea is the most ideal beverage to drink in the mornings. The anti-oxidants help flush out the toxins from the liver and also help perk up the Kupffer cells, which help in fighting disease causing pathogens.

### Dandelion tea

Dandelion is a weed, and has several healing properties. Dandelion greens can be consumed to help clean the liver. They can be cooked and eaten or the roots can be juiced. Another effective way of administering dandelion is by drinking dandelion tea. You can buy dandelion tea bags, which contain just the right amount of dried dandelion roots.

## Olive oil

There are many detox diet that ask you to drink olive oil daily, to decrease the chances of gallstones. But rather than drinking olive oil, you can definitely use it for your cooking purposes. Olive oil has many health properties, so it is better to choose olive oil instead of some other fat. Although oils such as olive and flax seed do not directly help the liver get rid of toxins, they work by absorbing the harmful chemicals before they reach the liver. They make for a good absorbent base, which absorb all the harmful toxins that can make the liver go into over drive. When you are using olive oil for cooking, make sure you do not over heat the oil, because by doing that the healthy good properties of the oil is lost. Use olive oil in salad dressings, to enhance the flavor of the salad.

## Aloe Vera juice

Aloe Vera leaf juice is extremely helpful in cleaning out the liver. It contains lots of chlorophyll and the sticky substance inside the leaf contains enzymes that help bind with the molecules of the toxins and transport them out of the body. Juiced Aloe Vera works best and you can add turmeric powder and honey to add leverage to the effects of the plant.

## *Contraindications for liver detox*

Liver detoxification should not be done by those individuals who already suffer from previous illnesses, as it is not safe for everyone. Detoxification includes a strict diet plan, which may be difficult to follow at the beginning. People who undergo detox may also experience symptoms like fatigue, weakness, nausea and headache. These symptoms occur due to the sudden change in eating habits of the individuals. If the symptoms are more aggressive, it is better you consult your physician regarding this, before continuing the detox process further. Here is a list of people who should not undergo detoxification:

- Pregnant and lactating mother
- People who suffer from heart disease.
- Individuals who are suffering from cancer.
- People who already have an active liver disease.
- The once who are diagnosed with diabetes and hypothyroidism.
- Individuals who are recovering from a surgery.
- Individuals who are below 18 years of age
- Individuals who are underweight.

## *Emotions and Food*

Emotions are an essential part of the detox plan. There are many individuals in the world for which food doesn't satisfy the physical hunger, but to satisfy their emotional need. You need to ask this question to yourself.

Why do you start to overeat after a period of starving? This is because your body is deprived of food, and is already into a state of depression, so when you tend to see food all of a sudden after days of starving, you naturally tend to eat more.

While undergoing detox, an individual may notice many emotional changes. This is because cleansing occurs both on mental and physical level. Many emotional toxins like fear, anxiety and stress are released when you detox the body. When you have such an emotional craving, try to understand your body, don't just think about food.

## *Try to identify your hunger: true or emotional*

The hunger sensation felt during the detox, might not be the true hunger feeling. It is necessary for one to keep attention on these sensations of hunger. Try to identify the exact need of your body at that moment. Ask yourself, what are you exactly feeling?

What is it, is it loneliness, boredom, sadness, anxiety? Figure out what is the true feeling, name it; do not replace it by food. This will help you in distinguishing between your true hunger and emotional hunger. This distinction will further help you to overcome your unnecessary food cravings and weight gain.

### *True hunger –*

- Arises gradually
- There is no overeating, you stop as soon as you are full
- Not necessary to be fulfilled at that particular moment
- You feel good after you are done with eating

### *Emotional hunger-*

- Arises suddenly
- Craving for a particular food
- There is over eating, you keep eating even when you are full.
- You feel guilty and shameful after eating

Emotional hunger tips- Drink a lot of water to curb your hunger; also green tea is a good option. Hydrate yourself; it helps to keep your bowels moving and eliminates toxins.

Try to concentrate on something else except for food.

Get up and go for a walk. Involve yourself in some activity and keep yourself moving.

### *Importance of breakfast*

"Eat breakfast like a king, lunch like a prince, and dinner like a pauper."

It is very important for your body to get a hearty breakfast in the morning, especially after the fasting window of about 10 to 12 hours. You give enough rest to your digestive system and breakfast is the time your liver should be active.

Breakfast should always be healthy and balanced. It should contain good amount of proteins and fats that helps to stimulate the liver in the morning by restoring the glycogen levels in the body. The liver when stimulated in the morning, functions normally throughout the day. Skipping of breakfast leads to a lot of negativity, decreased energy levels, slows down the metabolism and thus results in decreased liver functions.

### *Daily bowel movements*

When you are undergoing a detox, it is necessary for you to eliminate the trash out of your body. This trash contains a lot of toxins in it, and has to be eliminated regularly, so that the body does not reabsorb the toxins back into your system. If the body reabsorbs the toxins back into the system, the burden on the liver will increase.

When you don't remove the trash from your house, it will start to pile up, attract flies and then create a problem for you. The same implies to the body, if you do not evacuate everyday waste from your body, it will start to pile up in the body and give us problems later on in life.

Sometimes your bowel movements will increase when you are doing a detox, it could be 3 times a day, there is nothing to worry in it, is just that your internal system is going through a cleansing session. There are times when you may be constipated. If you are constipated here are few easy tips that you can follow to resolve it-

**Hydrate yourself**- drink enough water in the day, ideally you should drink about 4-5 liters of water a day. Hydrating yourself helps in digestion and clearing the bowels.

**Food rich in fiber**- include green leafy vegetables and fruits in your meals; they are a very good source of fiber. Luke warm water with lemon is also very helpfully in curbing constipation.

**Move yourself**- Walk and do some exercises. Basic yoga is also great and helps in relieving constipation.

### *Window period*

It is very true that our body is just like a machine, but yes it also needs enough rest, after working for the whole day. It needs rest to prepare itself for the next day too. You just cannot keep working all day long without resting. Your body gets exhausted over a period of time.

Digestion is one of the most important and energy consuming function of the body. If your body is continuously busy in digestion during the detox, then there is no time and energy left for the body for deep cleansing.

The body needs a window period of twelve hours. After consuming your evening meal, the body needs a twelve-hour window period before you have your first meal of the day. That is if you are eating your evening meal at 7 pm, you should consume your breakfast at 7 am or later.

Your body needs at least eight hours for accomplishing the process of digestion and then needs another four hours for deep cleanse.

If you have meals late at nights, and then eat early again the next day, your body does not get the time and opportunity to clean your system.

So avoid eating late at night, try to eat before 8 pm in the night for proper digestion. It is okay if you have water during this twelve hours window period.

# Chapter 7: Design Your Own Diet Plan For Detox

It is not very easy to incorporate all these food products in our daily diet all together at once. But make sure that you slowly start shifting your diet to a healthy one, by at least including one of these food products in your daily diet meal plan. It will definitely help you flush out those extra laded toxins of your body, making your body more fit and healthy.

Design your own diet detox plan, according to your taste and comfort. Initially it will be a little difficult for you to follow it sincerely and regularly, but as you become use to it you will start to enjoy your food. By doing little by little you are helping your liver to remove the toxins of the body, and prevent its further damage.

Individuals can opt for liver detox plan, according to their needs and capability. There are liver detox plans that can be followed for 6 months and even up to one year. These long plans are very monotonous and difficult to follow, therefore it is better to include these food products in your daily meal so that you can enjoy your meals without having to get stuck in a circle of detox and diets.

Create your own recipes. But make sure that all the ingredients that you use are on the approved list of food, for detox.

To make your detox journey easier, I have listed a few recipes that can help you with you liver detox.

# Chapter 8: Refreshing Juice Recipes

### Red Beetroot Energy Boosting Juice

**Ingredients**

- 2 beetroots
- 1 ½ carrots
- 2 handfuls of parsley
- ½ piece of ginger

**Method**

1. Thoroughly wash all the ingredients.
2. Parboil the beetroots, remember do not overcook the beetroots as they might lose all the nutrients.
3. Blend all the ingredients in a blender, and remove the juice in a glass.
4. Garnish it with some parsley leaves.
5. Refrigerate the juice and enjoy it chilled.

## *Mixed Berry Shake*

### Ingredients

- 2 cups frozen mixed berries, blueberries, raspberries, and cranberries
- 3-4 dates, deseeded
- 1 giant bunch of spinach
- 1 tablespoon hemp seeds
- 1 cup coconut water

### Method

1. Mix the berries, spinach, dates and hemp seeds in a blender, and blend until creamy.
2. Add coconut water to this and blend again.
3. Serve chilled.

## *Detoxifying Dandelion Shake*

### Ingredients

- 2 cups dandelion greens
- 3 cups coconut water
- 1 cup strawberries cut into pieces
- 1 cup frozen peach
- 1 tablespoon flax seeds
- ½ cup yogurt

### Method

1. Put the dandelion greens, strawberries, frozen peach and flax seeds into a blender and blend it.
2. Add coconut milk and yogurt to the blender and mix it again.
3. Remove the smoothie in a glass and serve cool.

## *Green Spinach Smoothie*

### Ingredients

- 2 handful bunch of spinach
- 2 lime, deseed, sliced and juiced.
- 1 cucumber
- 1 lemon, peeled and juiced
- Ice cubes, as per required

### Method

1. Thoroughly wash the spinach.
2. Blend all the ingredients in the juicer until smooth.
3. Add some crushed ice and sip on your chilled smoothie.

## *Apple Cinnamon Smoothie*

### Ingredients

- 2 frozen apples, cut and diced into small pieces
- 1 cup Greek yogurt
- ½ teaspoon cinnamon powder
- 1/2 teaspoon flax seeds

### Method

1. Put all the ingredients in a blender and give it a mix.
2. Pour the smoothie in a glass and serve chilled.

## *Strawberry and Mint Smoothie*

### Ingredients

- 2 cups fresh strawberries, the greens removed, washed and chopped roughly
- 1 cup yogurt
- 2-3 peppermint leaves
- 7-8 ice cubes
- ½ cup almond milk

### Method

1. Blend the strawberries properly in a mixer and make a thick puree.
2. To this, add the yogurt, mint leaves, crushed ice and almond milk and blend until the juice is smooth.
3. Pour it in a glass, and drink up whenever you feel hungry.

# Chapter 9: Healthy Salad Recipes

*Greek salad*

**Ingredients**

- 2 tomatoes, diced
- 1 chilled cucumber, peeled and diced
- 3-4 green olives cut in halves
- 1 cup green cabbage, shredded
- 1 small red onion, peeled and thinly sliced

**For the dressing**

- 2 tablespoons olive oil
- 1 garlic, peeled and minced
- 2 tablespoons lemon juice
- ¼ teaspoon black pepper

- Salt to taste
- Cilantro for garnishing

**Method**

1. Mix tomatoes, cucumbers, olives, cabbage and red onion in a large bowl.
2. Now in a small bowl, mix olive oil, lemon juice, garlic, pepper and salt until they mix together completely.
3. Pour the dressing over the fresh vegetables, and toss well.
4. Top it with some cilantro and serve.

# Roasted Squash and Asparagus Salad (topped with avocado dressing)

## Ingredients

- 1 cup butternut squash, peeled and diced
- 4-5 asparagus sticks
- Salt to taste
- For the dressing
- 2 ripe avocados, peeled and chopped
- 3 spring onions, use only the greens, finely chopped
- 2 tablespoon lemon juice
- Water as needed
- 1 small piece of ginger, peeled and roughly chopped
- Sea salt to taste
- 1 teaspoon apple cider vinegar

## Method

1. Heat a pan and lightly roast the butternut squash. Make sure you don't burn them because they will give you a bitter taste.

2. Now blanch the asparagus in water for 2-3 minutes, remember don't overcook them. When they are done place them under cold water, so that they retain their beautiful color and also the process of further cooking stops.

3. Keep aside the roasted squash and blanched asparagus, sprinkle little salt over it,

4. Now for the dressing, add avocados, spring onions, ginger and lemon juice into a blender and blend it.

5. Add little water to this dressing to get the perfect consistency and blend again. Now season the dressing with salt and apple cider vinegar. Mix all the ingredients properly.

6. Now add the dressing over the vegetables, and serve.

This salad is a complete source of nutrients and proteins. The combination of softened squash and crispy asparagus is unique and textural.

## *Frozen Cabbage Slaw*

### Ingredients

- 2 cups red cabbage, washed and finely chopped in length
- 1 medium red shallot, peeled and thinly sliced
- 1 small green bell pepper, deseeded and chopped in length

### For the dressing

- 1 cup yogurt
- 1 teaspoon freshly ground black pepper
- 2 teaspoons mixed herbs
- 2 tablespoons lemon juice
- 1 teaspoon olive oil
- ¼ teaspoon red chili powder
- Salt to taste
- Water as needed

### Method

1. Mix the cabbage, sliced shallots and capsicum together in a bowl.
2. Take a bowl, add some yogurt and start whisking it. Add olive oil to the yogurt and keep whisking until they incorporate.

3. Add lemon juice, salt, black pepper, chilli powder and mixed herbs and mix it again. Pour some water in this mixture, so that you get a proper dressing consistency.

4. Toss the vegetables and the dressing together and refrigerate. Serve chilled

## *Raw Vegetables and Fruit Salad*

**Ingredients-**

- 3-4 crunchy lettuce leaves, iceberg or arugula
- 1 medium sized tomato, thinly sliced
- 1 cucumber, peeled and chopped length wise
- 5-6 cherry tomatoes cut into halves
- 1 cup raspberries
- 1 cup blueberries
- Salt to taste
- 1 tablespoon lemon juice
- 2-3 basil leaves
- ¼ teaspoon chia seeds

**Method**

1. Take a bowl and mix the tomatoes, cucumbers, cherry tomatoes and the berries together.
2. Add to this mixture a ½ teaspoon of salt and lemon juice, and toss them together.
3. Take a plate and place the lettuce over it, and then the mixture of vegetables and fruits.
4. Garnish it with some basil leaves and chia seeds, and serve.

## *Peach, Avocado and Nut Salad*

### Ingredients-

- 3 ripe peaches cut in to small sized chunks
- 2 ripe avocados cut into small sized chunks
- 1 tablespoon lemon juice
- ¼ tablespoon walnuts
- 1 tablespoon chia seeds
- 2 tablespoon cilantro finely chopped

### Method

1. Toast the walnuts in a pan over low heat until they turn golden brown. Cool the nuts and roughly chop them and set aside.
2. Cut the peaches and avocados into same small sized chunks.
3. Add the toasted walnuts over the fruits.
4. Squeeze lemon juice over the mixture and toss until they combine well.
5. Add to the mixture chia seeds and finely chopped cilantro, and give it another toss and serve.

# Chapter 10: Soups

*Cauliflower and Carrot Bisque*

**Ingredients**

- 1 large cauliflower head, cut into pieces
- 2 tablespoon extra-virgin olive oil
- 1 medium onion, peeled and roughly chopped
- 1 carrot stick, peeled and chopped
- 2 cloves garlic, peeled and minced
- 4 cups vegetable stock
- 1 cup almond milk
- 2-3 fresh thyme sprigs
- 2 tablespoon lemon juice
- Salt to taste

- ½ teaspoon black pepper

**Method**

1. In a large saucepan, heat the olive oil over medium heat and sauté the garlic until it turns golden brown.

2. Add diced onions to the pan and cook it for 4-5 minutes, until they turn translucent and tender

3. Now add the cauliflower heads, diced carrots and a pinch of salt to the pan and keep stirring for 5 minutes continuously.

4. Add the vegetable stock and fresh thyme sprigs and cover the saucepan with a lid and let it simmer for 12-15 minutes, until the cauliflower and carrots are tender. Remember to simmer on low heat.

5. Take the pan off the heat and let the mixture cool. Now blend the mixture in a blender until smooth.

6. Add this pureed soup back into the saucepan and simmer it on low heat.

7. Add almond milk, salt, black pepper and lemon juice to the soup and stir well.

8. Garnish it with few sprigs of parsley and serve hot.

## Green Spinach Soup

**Ingredients**

- 2 cups freshly chopped spinach
- 1 onion, finely diced
- 2 garlic cloves, minced
- 1 small piece of ginger, peeled and juiced
- 1 and 1/2 cup of broccoli
- 2 tablespoon of olive oil
- 3 cups of vegetable broth
- 3 ribs of celery, finely chopped
- Salt to taste
- ½ teaspoon of freshly ground white pepper
- 1 tablespoon lemon juice

**Method**

1. Heat olive oil in a pan on medium heat. Add the freshly minced garlic to the hot oil, sauté it for a few minutes, until it turns golden brown.
2. Now add the chopped onions to the pan and cook for 3 minutes.
3. Add spinach, broccoli, parsley, celery and ginger to the pan. Mix all the ingredients properly.
4. Now add 3 cups of vegetable broth in it.

5. Cover the pan with the lid, and let the soup simmer for 15 minutes.

6. Now take off the pan from the heat, and the mixture aside to cool down. Pour all the mixture in a food processor and puree it.

7. Now pour the soup into a bowl and season it with salt, pepper and lemon juice.

## *Creamy Winter Beetroot Soup*

**Ingredients**

- 3 medium sized beetroots
- 2 shallots, peeled and diced
- Sea salt, to taste
- 2 garlic cloves, peeled and roughly chopped
- ½ ripe avocado, peeled and diced
- 1 cup of fresh coconut milk
- 1 tablespoon of apple cider vinegar
- ½ cup fresh parsley

**Method**

1. Peel the beetroot and cut them into halves.
2. Add the beetroots, shallots and garlic in a steamer filled with one inch water and steam all the vegetables until tender. If you don't have a steamer, you can fill one inch of water in a pot, place all the vegetables in the water, cover the lid and steam it.
3. Now blend all the ingredients in the blender, along with the leftover steaming liquid in the pot.
4. Add apple cider vinegar and parsley.
5. Pour enough coconut milk and blend together, to develop a smooth creamy consistency.
6. Season the soup with sea salt.
7. Garnish the soup with diced avocados and serve.

## *Carrot and Avocado Chilled Soup*

### Ingredients

- 3 cups roughly chopped carrots
- 1 medium sized shallot, peeled and quartered
- 2 cups ripe avocado
- Sea salt to taste
- 1 lime, peeled and juiced
- 5-6 hemp seeds
- Few mint leaves

### Method-

1. Place the carrots and shallot pieces in a pan, which is filled with 1-inch water.
2. Steam these vegetables for 5-6 minutes until they are done.
3. Remove the cooked vegetables from the pan and allow them to cool at room temperature.
4. Now pour the carrots and shallots in a blender and puree them.
5. Also add the avocado, hemp seeds, mint leaves and lime juice to it, and give it another mix, blend until you get a smooth consistency. If you feel that the soup is too thick, simply add little water to it, until you have the consistency that you want.
6. Season the soup with some sea salt as per your taste. Place the soup in the refrigerator to get chilled for 3-4 hours.
7. Enjoy the soup with a salad.

## Red Lentil and Vegetable Stew

### Ingredients

- 3 tablespoon olive oil
- 1 large onion, peeled and finely chopped
- 2 cloves of garlic, peeled and finely minced
- 1 small piece of ginger, peeled and finely minced
- 2 cups red lentils
- 2 cups chicken broth
- 1 cups chicken broth
- 2 tablespoon ground cumin powder
- 1 tablespoon ground coriander seeds
- Salt to taste
- 2 tablespoons lemon juice
- 2 tablespoons cilantro, finely chopped for garnishing

### Method-

1. Heat a soup pot over medium high flame and allow the olive oil to heat.
2. Add the onions in the pot when the oil reaches the appropriate temperature; cook them until they turn soft and translucent.
3. When the onions start to soften add finely minced ginger and garlic in the pan and cook until you get the fragrance.

4. Now add the freshly ground cumin powder, coriander powder and black pepper and stir well.

5. Reduce the heat and add coconut milk, cook for 5-6 minutes.

6. Now add the chicken stock and red lentils, and keep stirring to avoid the lentils from sticking at the sides of the pot.

7. When the lentils start to cook you will notice that the stew is thickening, add little water if required.

8. Cool down the mixture and blend the puree until smooth.

9. Add salt and lemon juice for seasoning, and garnish it with some finely chopped cilantro and serve warm.

# Chapter 11: Exercise And Yoga For Liver Cleanse

Regular exercise can help keep the entire body healthy, both internally and externally. Exercise helps in maintaining both physical as well as mental health. Exercise physically keeps you fit, healthy and energetic and mentally is keeps your mind calm, fresh and relaxed. It also helps in fighting daily stress.

There are several routines that you can follow in order to help cleanse the liver naturally.

Some of these exercises are mentioned and explained below but it is important to note that they do not necessarily, independently help in the process of cleansing and will require the doer to follow a strict diet regime in tandem with these exercises in order to reap their benefits.

It is also important to do at least 30 minutes to 1 hour of these exercises on a daily basis in order to see results.

- Cardio
- Yoga

### *Cardio*

You can do 30 minutes of cardio for 4 days in a week and incorporate the likes of cycling and swimming. They help the liver kick start their functioning and also prevent the building up of internal toxins by reducing stress.

### *Yoga*

Yoga moves are great to help cleanse the liver. They help your body get into positions, which allow your internal organs to have a good massage. They can literally squeeze out the toxins like squeezing out water from a sponge.

The following are some of the most beneficial yoga moves for you to adopt in order to cleanse your liver.

Remember do not push yourself too much into a yoga pose, if you are unable to do it. It will take time for you to attain proper posture; daily practice will help you improve slowly.

**Cat cow pose**

The cat cow pose is easy to perform and helps expand and contract the liver muscles.

To perform: - Place palms and knees on the mat such that your stomach is parallel to the floor.

Slowly bend forward while inhaling to resemble a cow and then arch your back upwards like a cat would.

Release and go to neutral position. Repeat 5 times.

**Chair twists**

Chair twists are great to massage the liver. They work on both the right and the left lobes and give the liver a good work out.

To Perform: - Stand straight with hands out stretched in front of you. Then fold hands as if to make a Namaste and pretend like you are sitting on an imaginary chair.

Now slowly turn you upper torso towards the right and hold pose. Come back to neutral and repeat on the other side.

**High-lunge twist**

To perform: - Start by standing straight with arms by your side.

Now place your right foot forward and push your left foot backwards. Twist upper torso and spread out arms such that your right arm lies parallel to your right thigh and left arm to left calf. Hold pose for a couple of seconds and release. Repeat on other side.

**Supine twist**

To perform: - Sleep on the floor with arms stretched on either side and legs joined.

Now slowly lift and place the right leg towards the left side such that it is perpendicular to the left leg. Hold pose and return to neutral pose.

Repeat pose with the other leg.

**Cobra pose**

To perform: - Lie down with your stomach on the floor and arms by your side.

Now place both palms facing down under your chest and slowly lift yourself up. Lift only the upper torso with the lower torso remaining glued to the floor. Lift head and look upwards.

Hold the pose for a couple of minutes and repeat 5 times.

**Downward facing three legged dog**

To perform: - Sleep with your stomach on the floor.

Assume the cobra pose and slowly lift your posterior upwards. Balance your body with your palms and toes.

Now slowly lift your left leg upwards and hold pose. Go back to neutral and repeat with right leg.

## Forward fold with twist

To perform: - Stand straight with arms to your side and slowly bend forward so as to touch your toes.

Then twist to the left and place your right palm on your outer left ankle and lift your right hand straight upwards.

Hold pose for a couple of seconds and release.

Repeat the pose with the other leg. Repeat 2 times each.

## Boat pose

To perform: - Sit straight with legs stretched out and a straight back.

Now stretch out hands such that they are parallel to your legs.

Now lift legs to a 45-degree angle and lift your arms such that your fingers point at your feet.

Hold pose for a couple of minutes and release.

## Shoulder stand

To perform: - Sleep on the floor with arms to your side.

Now slowly lift legs upwards to a 90 degrees and lift up lower back.

Support lower back with your palms and fingers and hold pose. Release and return to neutral.

Repeat 2 times.

## Bridge pose

To perform: - Sleep with back on the floor and legs folded such that knees point to the roof and hands to your side.

Now slowly lift your lower torso upwards and make sure your feet don't leave the floor.

Hold the pose for a couple of seconds and return to neutral.

These are some of the best yoga poses that you can perform and cleanse your liver.

# Chapter 12: Foods To Avoid

When you decide to detox your liver, you will have to abstain from the consumption of certain foods, which can prevent you from garnering any positive results.

## *Alcohol*

Alcohol is your liver's worst enemy. Alcohol can be too burdensome for the liver to process and hitting it with heavy amounts can lead to diseases such as fatty liver disease and cirrhosis.

It is extremely crucial to avoid drinking absolutely any form of alcohol while on the detox diet.

## *Gluten rich foods*

Foods rich in gluten such as wheat can burden your liver. Breaking down complex gluten molecules can take a lot of effort, which can slow down your liver's healing capacity.

It is therefore advisable to avoid as much gluten as possible while you undergo a liver cleansing.

### Smoking

When you smoke, you end up damaging all internal parts of your body including your liver.

One of the most dangerous of results of smoking is the decreased capacity of the red blood cells to carry oxygen to the various parts of your body. That means the liver does not get enough blood coming in for it to work optimally.

It is therefore crucial to not smoke while on the diet and to stop smoking in general.

### Junk food

Packaged and processed foods such as cereals, sodas, biscuits, chocolates etc. are laden with harmful artificial flavors that can damage your liver.

They contain just so much impurities that the liver becomes incapable of clearing all of it out and ultimately slows it down.

It is therefore imperative to avoid processed and junk foods while on the liver cleansing routine.

### Sugars

Sugary foods such as chocolates, biscuits, cakes, sweets and other sugar filled snacks can be extremely taxing for the liver. It can convert sugars to glycogen and store it, yes but there is a limit to it. Over burdening it will lead to insulin resistance and the liver will stop working optimally.

Therefore it is advisable to stave off the consumption of sugary foods while on the liver detox diet.

### Coffee and tea

Coffee and tea contains caffeine, which is not easily broken down. The liver has to put in a lot of effort to break down the molecules of caffeine and separate it. Dairy products also prove to be too heavy for the liver.

If you cannot give up on your beverages then you can consume just half a cup in the mornings and avoid consuming it at night.

## *Pesticides and artificial fertilizers*

Buy your groceries from places where vegetables and fruits are grown organically. Try locating an organic market and buy your produce from there.

If you cannot find any such place then make sure you thoroughly wash your vegetables and fruits in preferably vinegar water to wash off as much chemicals as possible, before cooking and consuming them.

## *Monosodium glutamate*

Better known as MSG, this chemical is most popular in Chinese dishes and as a preservative. MSG can over excite your liver cells causing them to tire out very easily.

Therefore avoid packaged soups, salad seasonings, frozen desserts etc.

## *Starch and carbs*

Starchy foods and foods laden with carbs like rice, bread, pasta and potatoes can lead to insulin resistance. This resistance can cause the liver to function abnormally.

## *Trans-fats*

Trans-fats can come in the way of your body's ability to burn fat and also slow down the functioning of your liver. They can thicken the bile, which causes indigestion and loose bowels.

## *Red meats*

Red meats can be too heavy for your liver. They are tougher to break down and might impede your liver's capacity to digest food.

Also if you still wish to continue eating meat, try to consume meat of those animals that are grass fed, rather than those which have been fed on antibiotics and hormones.

It is therefore important to avoid red meats while on the liver cleansing diet.

## *Avoid stale food*

Always make it a habit to eat fresh food. Stale food when left for overnight or even for many days starts to develop bacteria's and toxins in it. The food starts to decay, and so this taxes up the liver to filter more toxins from the body. So it is very essential to have fresh food that is cooked on every day basis.

## *Do not over eat*

Remember this one important thing: never overeat. Try to avoid overloading your digestive system with excess food. Over eating makes the action of digestion very sluggish and also decreases the metabolic activity, thus accumulating a large amount of food in the colon and also increases the toxins. It is necessary to keep a watch on the portion size that you consume.

Occasionally fast or just go on a liquid diet, giving your body a little break from the normal routine. Include healthy soups, fresh juice, green tea and water in your liquid diet. Overeating leads to congestion of the digestive system, which disturbs its normal function.

Always break your meals in small portions to avoid over loading at once. Make a habit of consuming six meals a day at regular intervals so that digestion takes place properly. Also chew your food properly do not just gulp down your food.

# Conclusion

In this book, we explored the various functions of the liver and understood how important it is for a person to maintain a clean liver in order to lead a healthy life.

We looked at the various foods that can be consumed in order to naturally cleanse the liver and promote its optimal functioning. Also we have talked on various food products one should avoid, while going through a liver detox.

We also saw the various exercises, which help in cleaning the organ and how alternate therapies are also available to help clean the liver.

This book provides you with various recipes so that you can enjoy your detox plan thoroughly.

We hope you had a good read and understood the steps that you must take to manually induce a liver cleansing process.

We thank you once again for giving this eBook, "Liver Detoxification" your time.

Happy cleansing!

## YOU MAY ENJOY MY OTHER BOOKS

DUKAN DIET: Four Phase Plan To Lose Weight FAST And FOREVER

smarturl.it/dukan

DETOX DIET CLEANSE: 7 Day Plan To Boost Energy and Change Your Life

hyperurl.co/detoxdiet

SUGAR: Shut Your Mouth To Sugar Addiction And Cravings

hyperurl.co/sugar

# RECOMMENDED READING

AUTOIMMUNE DISEASE ANTI-INFLAMMATORY DIET

smarturl.it/autoa

Crystals and Gemstones: Healing The Body Naturally

smarturl.it/crystala

HEALING: Heal Your Body Heal Your Life

smarturl.it/healingaa

NLP Subconscious Mind Power: Change Your Mind Change Your Life

hyperurl.co/NLP

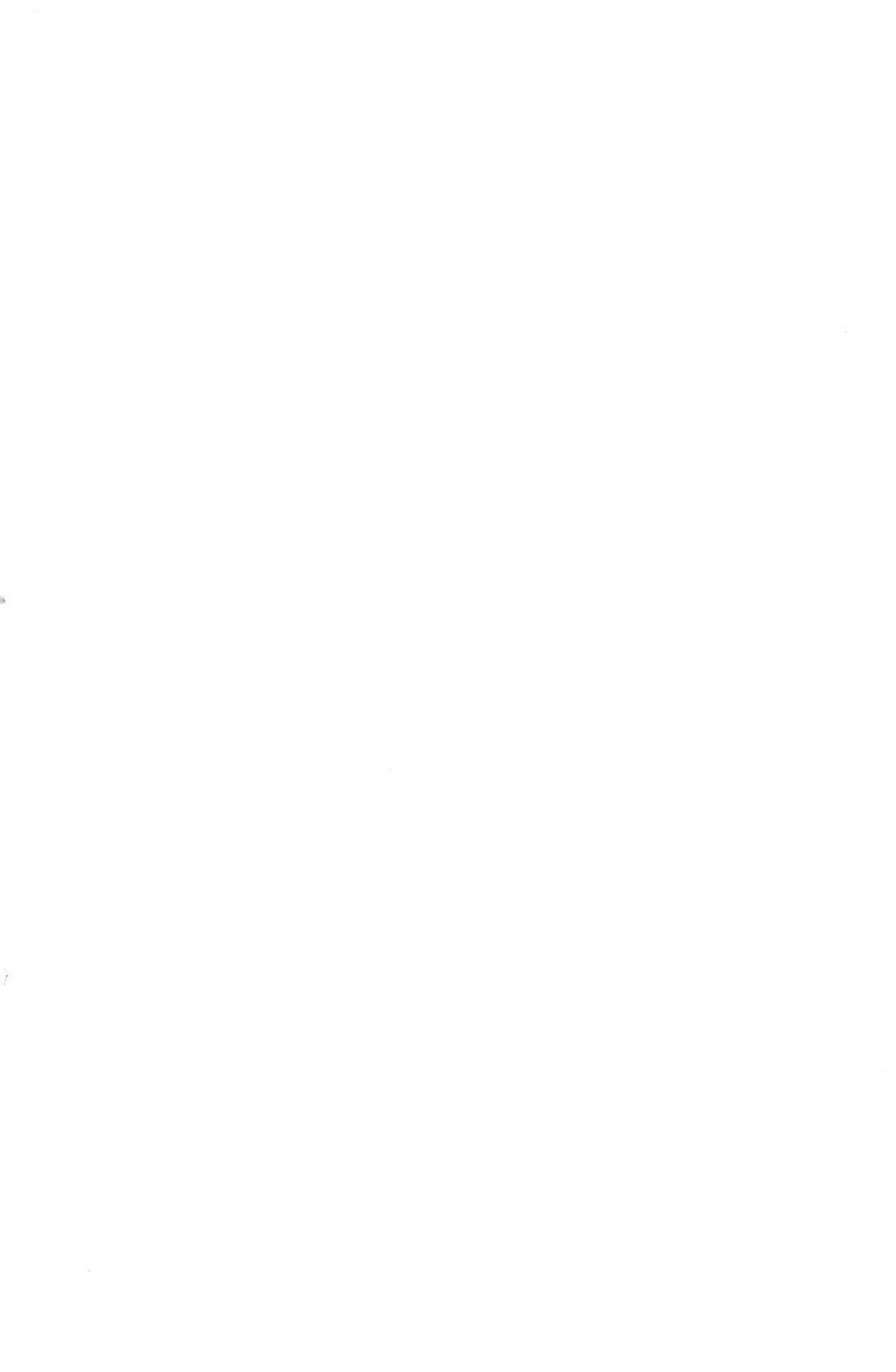

Made in the USA
Lexington, KY
18 November 2015